The Woodchopper Ab challenge

Functional Training for a Stronger Core

Helen Talbott

Disclaimer

The information contained in this book is for educational purposes only and is not intended to be a substitute for professional medical advice, diagnosis, or treatment. Always seek the advice of your physician or other qualified healthcare provider with any questions you may have regarding a medical condition.

The author and publisher disclaim any liability for any errors or omissions contained in this book and for any damages or losses incurred as a result of using the information provided.

Table of contents

About the Author

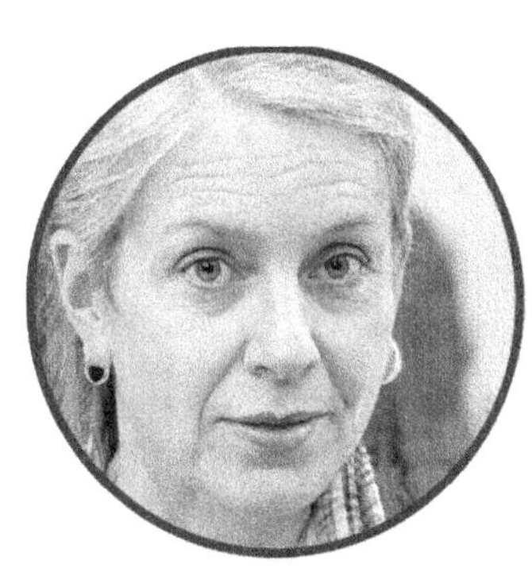

I'm Helen Talbott, a certified personal usetrainer and fitness enthusiast with a passion for empowering individuals to reach their health and wellness goals. Throughout my career, I've witnessed firsthand the transformative power of core strength, not just for aesthetics, but for overall well-being and peak performance.

My approach to fitness emphasizes **functional training**, focusing on exercises that mimic everyday movements and translate into real-life benefits. This philosophy is the cornerstone of **The Woodchopper Ab challenge** .

Why The Woodchopper Ab challenge ?

The woodchopper exercise, often overlooked, is a dynamic movement that engages a multitude of core muscles, promoting stability, power transfer, and rotational control. This challenge takes the woodchopper exercise as its foundation, building upon it with a variety of complementary exercises to create a **well-rounded core training challenge** .

What to Expect:

In this book, you'll discover:

- **The science behind core strength and its impact on overall health and fitness.**
- **A step-by-step guide to mastering the woodchopper exercise with proper form and technique.**
- **A diverse selection of core exercises, categorized by their target muscle groups and training goals.**
- **Sample workout routines tailored to various fitness levels and goals, from beginner to advanced.**

- **Nutritional guidance to support your core training journey and optimize results.**
- **Lifestyle tips to promote core health and stability beyond the gym.**

The Woodchopper Ab challenge is your guide to building a strong, functional core that not only looks good but also empowers you to move with confidence, prevent injuries, and achieve your fitness aspirations.

Let's embark on this journey together!

Introduction

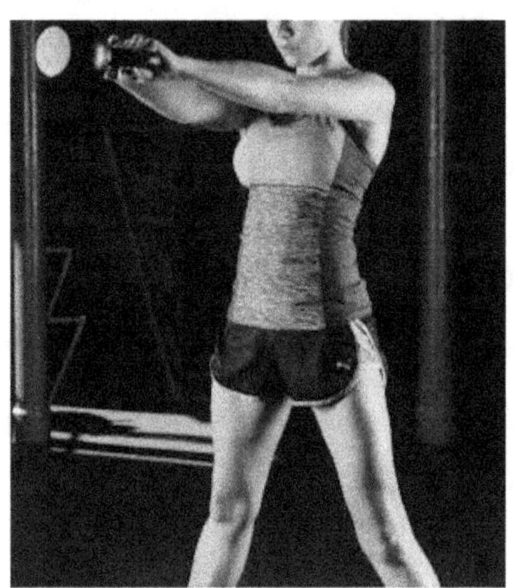

Welcome to the Woodchopper Ab Revolution

Have you ever dreamt of a core as strong and defined as a lumberjack's? Do you crave a midsection that not only looks good but also functions at its peak, allowing you to perform everyday activities with ease and power? Look no further than the **Woodchopper Ab challenge** , your ultimate guide to unlocking the full potential of your core through this dynamic and functional exercise.

This book is more than just a collection of exercises; it's a comprehensive challenge designed to transform your understanding of core training and empower you to achieve a stronger, healthier, and more functional you. We'll delve into the science of core strength, debunk myths about six-pack abs, and introduce you to the woodchopper exercise, a powerful movement that transcends aesthetics and targets the core in a way that translates into real-world benefits.

Why the Woodchopper?

The woodchopper isn't just another trendy exercise. It's a functional movement that mimics the rotational motion used in various everyday activities, from swinging a golf club to picking up groceries. By incorporating this exercise into your routine, you'll not only sculpt your abs but also:

- **Improve your functional strength and stability:** The woodchopper engages multiple muscle groups, including your obliques, transverse abdominis, and lower back, creating a strong and stable core that supports your entire body during daily activities.

- **Reduce your risk of injury:** A strong core plays a crucial role in maintaining proper posture and protecting your spine. The woodchopper strengthens the muscles that support your lower back, helping to prevent injuries and improve your overall well-being.

- **Enhance your athletic performance:** Whether you're a seasoned athlete or just starting your fitness journey, a strong core is essential for optimal performance. The woodchopper can help improve your balance, coordination, and power transfer, allowing you to perform at your best in any activity.

What to Expect from this challenge :

This challenge   is designed to cater to individuals of all fitness levels. Whether you're a beginner just starting your core training journey or a seasoned athlete looking to take your core strength to the next level, we've got you covered.

Here's what you can expect:

- **A comprehensive understanding of your core:** We'll break down the anatomy and function of your core muscles, helping you understand how they work together to create a strong and stable foundation.
- **Mastering the woodchopper exercise:** We'll provide a step-by-step guide to performing the woodchopper with perfect form, ensuring you maximize the benefits of this exercise while minimizing the risk of injury.
- **Building your personalized woodchopper ab challenge :** We'll offer sample workouts tailored to different fitness levels and goals, allowing you to customize your challenge and track your progress.
- **Beyond the woodchopper:** We'll explore additional core exercises that complement

the woodchopper, helping you build a well-rounded core training challenge .

- **Holistic approach to core development:** We understand that core strength goes beyond just exercise. We'll provide insights into the role of nutrition and lifestyle habits in supporting a healthy and strong core.

By the end of this challenge , you'll not only have a stronger and more defined core, but you'll also have gained a deeper understanding of its importance and how to maintain it for a lifetime of health and well-being. So, are you ready to unleash your inner lumberjack and embark on the **Woodchopper Ab Revolution**? Let's get started!

Welcome to the Woodchopper Ab challenge

Unleash Your Inner Lumberjack and Build a Stronger Core

Do you fantasize about possessing a core as powerful and defined as a seasoned lumberjack? Do you yearn for a midsection that not only boasts an aesthetic appeal but also functions optimally, allowing you to effortlessly navigate everyday tasks with strength and stability? Look no further than the **Woodchopper Ab challenge**, a comprehensive guide designed to unlock the full potential of your core through the dynamic and functional exercise known as the woodchopper.

This challenge transcends the realm of simply providing an assortment of exercises. It's a meticulously crafted journey designed to revolutionize your understanding of core training and empower you to achieve a state of enhanced strength, improved health, and a more functional you. We'll delve into the fascinating science of core strength, dispel the prevalent myths surrounding six-pack abs, and introduce you to the woodchopper, a potent movement that transcends mere aesthetics, targeting your core in a way that translates into tangible real-world benefits.

Why Embark on the Woodchopper Ab challenge ?

The woodchopper isn't simply another exercise that rides the fleeting wave of fitness trends. It's a functional movement that mirrors the rotational motion employed in a multitude of daily activities, ranging from the graceful swing of a golf club to the mundane task of picking up groceries. By incorporating this exercise into your routine, you'll not only sculpt a sculpted abdomen, but also:

- **Cultivate superior functional strength and stability:** The woodchopper engages a multitude of muscle groups, including your obliques, transverse abdominis, and lower back muscles, fostering a robust and stable core that acts as a central pillar of support for your entire body during everyday activities.

- **Minimize your risk of sustaining injuries:** A strong core plays a pivotal role in maintaining proper posture and safeguarding your spine. The woodchopper strengthens the muscles responsible for supporting your lower back, helping to prevent injuries and enhancing your overall well-being.
- **Elevate your athletic performance:** Regardless of whether you're a seasoned athlete or just embarking on your fitness journey, a robust core is fundamental to achieving optimal performance. The woodchopper can significantly improve your balance, coordination, and power transfer, enabling you to perform at your peak in any activity.

What Treasures Await You Within This challenge :

This challenge is meticulously crafted to cater to individuals of diverse fitness levels. Whether you're a novice just starting your core training journey or a seasoned athlete seeking to elevate your core strength to the next level, we've meticulously curated content to meet your needs.

Here's a glimpse of the invaluable knowledge and tools you'll acquire:

- **A comprehensive understanding of your core:** We'll embark on a voyage of discovery, delving into the anatomy and function of your core muscles. This journey will equip you with a profound understanding of how these muscles work synergistically to create a robust and stable foundation for your body.
- **Mastering the art of the woodchopper:** We'll provide a step-by-step, meticulously detailed guide on executing the woodchopper with flawless form. This

ensures you maximize the benefits of this exercise while minimizing the risk of injury.

- **Crafting your personalized woodchopper ab challenge :** We'll offer a variety of sample workouts specifically tailored to diverse fitness levels and goals. This empowers you to customize your challenge to seamlessly integrate into your routine and meticulously track your progress.

- **Beyond the realm of the woodchopper:** We'll venture beyond the woodchopper, exploring additional core exercises that complement this potent movement. This allows you to construct a well-rounded core training challenge that holistically addresses your core development needs.

- **A holistic approach to core development:** We acknowledge that core strength encompasses more than just exercise. We'll provide insightful guidance on the role of nutrition and essential lifestyle habits in fostering a healthy and robust core.

By the time you culminate this challenge , you'll not only possess a core that is stronger and more aesthetically pleasing, but you'll also have acquired a deeper comprehension of its significance and the strategies to maintain it for a lifetime of health and well-being. So, are you prepared to unleash your inner lumberjack and embark on the transformative journey of the **Woodchopper Ab challenge** ? Let's commence our quest for a stronger and more functional you!

What Awaits You in the Woodchopper Ab challenge

A Roadmap to Core Strength

The **Woodchopper Ab challenge** is not just another collection of exercises; it's a carefully designed roadmap leading you to a stronger, healthier, and more functional you. Here's what you can expect from this comprehensive challenge :

Unveiling the Core Mystery:

- **Demystifying Core Function:** We'll embark on a journey to understand your core beyond just six-pack abs. You'll learn about the intricate network of muscles that make up your core, their individual functions, and how they work together to create a stable and powerful foundation for your body.
- **Debunking the Six-Pack Myth:** We'll explore the truth behind the elusive six-pack abs and shift your focus towards

building a healthy and functional core, which is essential for overall well-being and performance.

Mastering the Art of the Woodchopper:

- **Step-by-Step Guide:** We'll take you through a detailed, step-by-step breakdown of the woodchopper exercise, ensuring you understand the proper form and technique to maximize its effectiveness and prevent injuries.
- **Variations and Progressions:** You'll discover various woodchopper variations tailored to different fitness levels and equipment availability. Whether you're a beginner or an advanced athlete, we'll guide you towards the most suitable variation. We'll also provide progressions to help you gradually increase the difficulty as you get stronger.

Crafting Your Personalized Journey:

- **Sample Workouts for Diverse Goals:** We offer a variety of sample workouts specifically designed for different fitness levels and goals. Whether you're aiming to build core strength, improve stability, or enhance rotational power, there's a challenge tailored for you.
- **Customization and Tracking:** The challenge empowers you to customize your workouts based on your preferences and schedule. We provide guidance on how to track your progress, allowing you to celebrate your achievements and stay motivated.

Expanding Your Core Training Arsenal:

- **Complementary Core Exercises:** We'll introduce you to a variety of exercises that complement the woodchopper, helping you build a well-rounded core training challenge that targets different muscle groups and movement patterns.
- **Building a Holistic Routine:** We recognize the importance of a holistic

approach to core development. We'll explore exercises that engage your core throughout your entire workout routine, maximizing its effectiveness.

Optimizing Your Core Development:

- **Nutritional Insights:** We'll delve into the role of proper nutrition in building and maintaining a strong core. You'll learn about essential nutrients and dietary strategies to support your core development goals.
- **Lifestyle Habits:** We'll discuss the impact of lifestyle habits like sleep and stress management on core health and provide practical tips to optimize these areas for improved results.

Beyond the challenge :

- **Maintaining Your Gains:** We'll equip you with the knowledge and tools to maintain your newfound core strength and stability in the long term, ensuring you reap the benefits throughout your life.

- **Continuing Your Core Journey:** We'll provide resources and recommendations to help you continue your core training journey beyond this challenge , allowing you to explore new exercises and further refine your core strength and functionality.

By embarking on the **Woodchopper Ab challenge** , you'll embark on a transformative journey towards a stronger, healthier, and more functional core. Remember, consistency and dedication are key to unlocking your full potential. So, are you ready to unleash your inner lumberjack and begin your core transformation? Let's chop our way to a stronger you!

Part 1

Understanding Your Core

Chapter 1

The Woodchopper

A Multifaceted Approach to Core Strength

While the quest for sculpted abs often dominates popular culture, a truly strong core encompasses far more than just aesthetics. The core, consisting of your abdominal muscles, lower back muscles, and obliques, acts as the central powerhouse of your body, responsible for stability, posture, and efficient movement. Enter the woodchopper exercise, a dynamic movement that transcends the realm of simply carving out six-pack abs, offering a multitude of benefits for building a robust and functional core.

Functional Strength and Stability: Unlike isolated exercises that target specific muscle groups, the woodchopper mimics a rotational movement pattern employed in various everyday activities. This translates to **functional strength**. As you perform the woodchopper, your core muscles work together to stabilize your spine and trunk, mimicking actions like swinging a golf club, throwing a ball, or simply picking up groceries. By strengthening these muscles, you improve your ability to perform daily tasks with ease and reduce the risk of injury from awkward movements.

Enhanced Balance and Coordination: The woodchopper challenges your body to maintain proper balance and coordination throughout the movement. This is because the exercise requires you to transfer weight from one leg to another while maintaining a stable torso and core. This translates to improved **balance and coordination** in everyday activities, reducing the risk of falls and enhancing your overall athletic performance.

Increased Power Transfer: The rotational motion of the woodchopper involves transferring power from your core to your limbs. This not only strengthens your core muscles but also improves your ability to **transfer power** efficiently. This translates to benefits in various sports like golf, tennis, and baseball, where efficient power transfer is crucial for optimal performance.

Reduced Risk of Lower Back Pain: A weak core can contribute to lower back pain, as the muscles aren't strong enough to properly support the spine. The woodchopper strengthens the muscles that support your lower back, improving **posture** and reducing the strain on your spine. This can significantly **reduce your risk of lower back pain**, especially when combined with proper form and technique.

Engages Multiple Muscle Groups: Unlike isolated core exercises that focus on a single muscle group, the woodchopper is a **compound exercise** that engages multiple muscle groups simultaneously. This includes your abs, obliques, lower back muscles, glutes, shoulders, and even your legs. By working multiple muscle groups, the woodchopper provides a more efficient workout, maximizing your time and effort.

Scalable for Different Fitness Levels: The beauty of the woodchopper lies in its **versatility**. You can adjust the difficulty based on your fitness level by using various weights, performing bodyweight variations, or altering the range of motion. This makes it suitable for beginners, advanced athletes, and everyone in between.

The woodchopper is not just another fad exercise; it's a potent tool for building a strong, functional, and healthy core. Its benefits extend far beyond aesthetics, offering functional strength, improved balance and coordination, enhanced power transfer, lower risk of injury, and engagement of multiple muscle groups. So, grab your metaphorical axe and prepare to chop your way to a stronger core, one rep at a time!

Key Core Muscles Targeted by the Woodchopper

The woodchopper exercise, often associated with chiseled abs, goes beyond mere aesthetics. It's a dynamic movement that orchestrates a symphony of core muscle engagement, promoting strength, stability, and power. Let's delve into the key core muscles targeted by the woodchopper, understanding their individual roles in this powerful exercise.

The Powerhouse Trio:

1. **Rectus Abdominis:** This is the oft-coveted "six-pack" muscle, lying vertically along the front of your abdomen. While the woodchopper doesn't directly target the rectus abdominis for flexion, it engages it isometrically, meaning the muscle contracts without changing length. This isometric contraction provides **stability and**

support to the spine throughout the movement.

2. **Obliques:** The woodchopper shines in targeting the obliques, the muscles that wrap around the sides of your torso. They are responsible for **rotation and lateral bending**. During the woodchopper, as you rotate your torso and diagonally bring your arm down, the **external obliques** on the opposite side contract to initiate the rotation. Additionally, the **internal obliques** on the same side contract to provide stability and control the movement.

3. **Transverse Abdominis (TVA):** Often referred to as the "deep core" muscle, the TVA acts like a natural internal corset, wrapping around your entire torso. While its contraction isn't directly visible, the woodchopper effectively engages the TVA. As you perform the exercise with proper form, the TVA **draws your belly button inwards**, creating **intra-abdominal pressure** that stabilizes

your spine and protects your internal organs.

Supporting Players:

Beyond the core muscles, the woodchopper also engages several other muscle groups that contribute to its effectiveness:

- **Lower Back Muscles:** The **erector spinae** and other muscles in your lower back work isometrically to maintain **spinal alignment** and **posture** throughout the movement.
- **Hip Flexors:** The **psoas major** and **iliacus** muscles in your hips engage to **initiate the movement** as you step forward and bring your torso down.
- **Glutes:** The **gluteus maximus** and **gluteus medius** work to **stabilize your pelvis** and **transfer power** from the lower body to the upper body during the rotation.
- **Shoulders:** The **rotator cuff muscles** in your shoulders stabilize the shoulder joint

and **control the arm movement** as you diagonally bring it down and then extend it upwards.

The Synergy:

The beauty of the woodchopper lies in its ability to **engage multiple muscle groups simultaneously**. This creates a **synergistic effect**, where each muscle group works together in harmony to achieve the desired movement. By strengthening these muscles, you not only build a stronger core but also improve your overall functional strength and stability.

The Takeaway:

The woodchopper isn't just an "ab exercise"; it's a multifaceted movement that targets a multitude of core muscles, along with supporting muscle groups. By understanding the roles of each muscle involved, you can appreciate the intricate choreography of the woodchopper and its potential to enhance your core strength, stability, and overall well-being.

Part 2

Chapter 2

Mastering the Woodchopper Exercise

A Step-by-Step Guide to Perfect Form

The woodchopper exercise, often associated with chiseled abs, offers far more than just aesthetics. It's a functional movement that strengthens and engages your core while improving stability and power transfer. However, proper form is crucial to maximize the benefits and minimize the risk of injury. Here's a step-by-step guide to performing the woodchopper with perfect form:

Equipment:

- Dumbbell (weight appropriate for your fitness level)

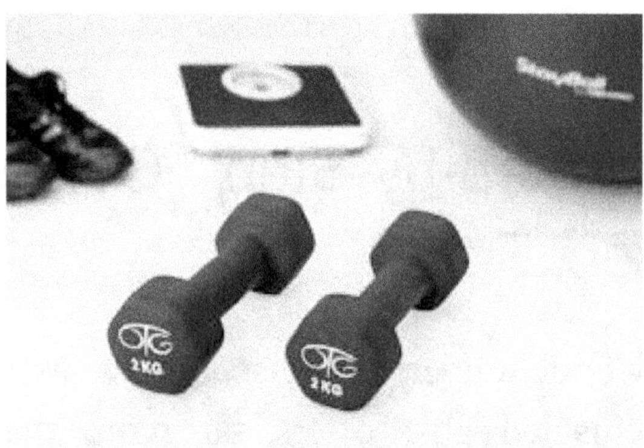

- Optional: Exercise mat (provides extra padding for your knees)

Starting Position:

1. Stand with your feet shoulder-width apart,
    core engaged, and back straight.

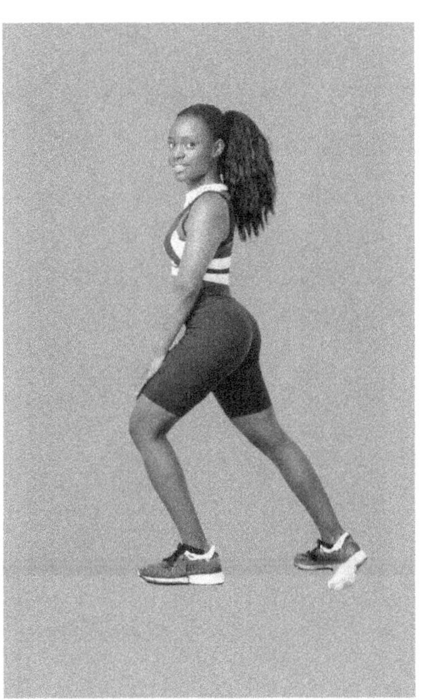

Hold the dumbbell in both hands, arms extended straight down in front of your thighs, palms facing your body.

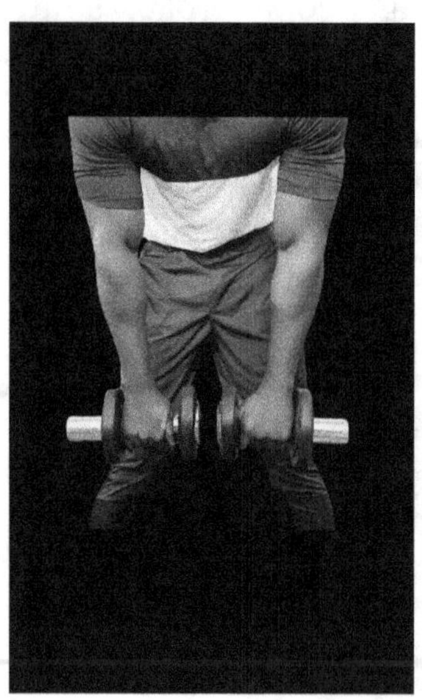

The Movement:

1. **Initiate the rotation:** Begin by rotating your torso **diagonally** towards the side **opposite** the hand holding the dumbbell. This is not a full torso twist; think of it as coiling your core muscles.

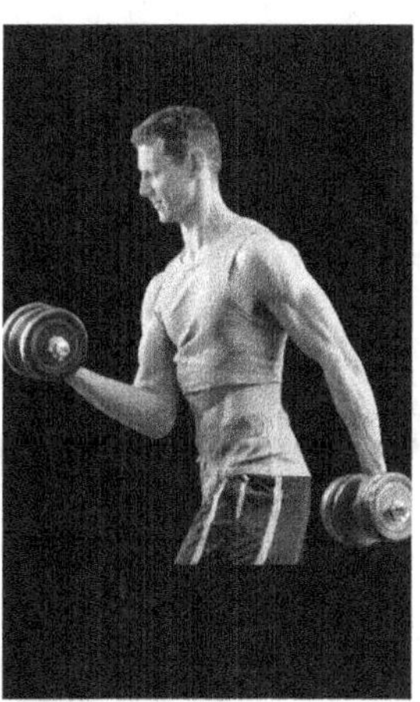

2. **Engage the legs:** As you rotate, **step forward** with the leg on the same side as the hand **holding** the dumbbell. This is a **lunge** position, with your front knee bent and your back knee slightly extended towards the ground.

3. **Chop the wood:** Simultaneously with the rotation and lunge, **lift** the dumbbell diagonally **upwards** across your body, as if chopping wood. The dumbbell should travel close to your torso, and your arm should be **slightly bent** at the elbow. Aim for the top of the dumbbell to reach the side of your chest, near your armpit.

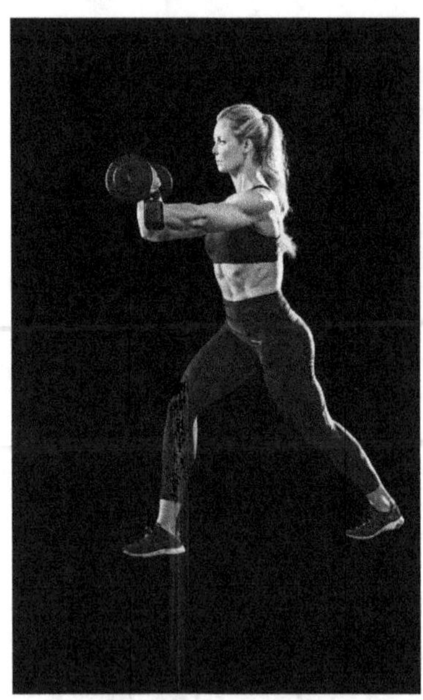

4. **Extend and return:** Fully extend your arm at the top of the movement,

maintaining your core engagement and a neutral spine. **Reverse** the movement by lowering the dumbbell back down diagonally across your body, returning to the starting position.

5. **Repeat:** Repeat the exercise for the desired number of repetitions, then switch sides and perform the same steps with the dumbbell held in the other hand.

Key Points for Perfect Form:

- **Maintain a neutral spine:** Keep your back straight and avoid excessive arching or rounding throughout the movement.
- **Engage your core:** Keep your core engaged throughout the entire movement, drawing your belly button inwards slightly. This provides stability and protects your lower back.
- **Focus on rotation, not just arm movement:** The primary movement should come from your core rotation, not just your arms lifting the weight.

- **Keep your shoulders stable:** Don't shrug your shoulders or allow them to round forward. Maintain a proud chest and engaged shoulder blades.
- **Controlled movement:** Perform the exercise in a controlled and deliberate manner, avoiding jerking or swinging motions.
- **Focus on your breath:** Breathe out as you lift the weight and inhale as you lower it.

Additional Tips:

- Start with a lighter weight to ensure proper form before increasing the weight.
- You can perform the woodchopper with bodyweight only (no dumbbell) for beginners.
- Focus on quality over quantity. It's better to perform fewer repetitions with good form than many repetitions with poor form.

- If you experience any pain, stop the exercise and consult a healthcare professional.

By following these steps and focusing on proper form, you can effectively utilize the woodchopper exercise to sculpt a strong and functional core, while minimizing the risk of injury and maximizing the benefits. Remember, consistency and proper technique are key to unlocking the full potential of this powerful exercise.

Exploring Variations of the Woodchopper Exercise

The woodchopper exercise, renowned for its ability to sculpt a strong and functional core, offers versatility beyond its seemingly straightforward execution. By incorporating various variations, you can cater to different fitness levels, target specific muscle groups, and keep your workouts challenging and engaging. Here, we delve into the diverse world of woodchopper variations, empowering you to tailor this exercise to your unique needs and goals.

Variations for Level Progression:

- **Bodyweight Woodchopper:** This variation is ideal for beginners or those new to the exercise. It allows you to focus on mastering the proper form and movement pattern without the added weight of a dumbbell. Once comfortable, you can progress to weighted variations.

- **Medicine Ball Woodchopper:** This variation adds a dynamic element to the exercise, challenging your core stability and coordination. Hold a medicine ball in both hands instead of a dumbbell and perform the woodchopper movement as usual. The increased instability of the medicine ball requires your core to work harder to maintain control and stability.
- **Cable Woodchopper:** Utilize a cable machine for a smooth and controlled resistance. Attach a handle to the cable and perform the woodchopper movement with your torso facing the machine. This variation allows for precise control of the weight and resistance throughout the exercise.

Variations for Muscle Group Emphasis:

- **Single-Leg Woodchopper:** Elevate the challenge and target your core stabilizers further by performing the woodchopper on one leg at a time. Start with a sturdy stance on one leg and perform the woodchopper movement, ensuring you maintain good balance and core engagement throughout.

- **Russian Twist Woodchopper:** This variation combines the rotational movement of the Russian twist with the diagonal chop of the woodchopper. Start in a standing position, holding a dumbbell in both hands. Perform a diagonal twist towards one side, bringing the dumbbell down towards your hip, then twist back to center and repeat on the other side.

- **Reverse Woodchopper:** This variation targets your core from a different angle, placing emphasis on the lower back and gluteal muscles. Stand with your back to the cable machine or hold a dumbbell behind your back. Perform the woodchopper movement in reverse, starting with the dumbbell near your hip and chopping it upwards across your body diagonally.

Variations for Equipment Adaptation:

- **Barbell Woodchopper:** Utilizing a barbell adds significant weight and challenges your core strength further. However, it's crucial to ensure proper form and technique to avoid injury. This variation is recommended for advanced individuals comfortable handling heavier weights.
- **Kettlebell Woodchopper:** The unique design of a kettlebell allows for a different grip and movement pattern compared to a dumbbell. Hold the kettlebell by the handle and perform the woodchopper movement, focusing on maintaining a neutral spine and core engagement.
- **TRX Woodchopper:** Utilize suspension straps like TRX for a challenging and bodyweight-based variation. Adjust the angle of the straps to find a suitable difficulty level and perform the woodchopper movement, focusing on core

engagement and maintaining proper body position.

Remember:

- Choose variations that suit your fitness level and goals.
- Always prioritize proper form over heavier weights.
- Don't hesitate to seek guidance from a certified trainer or fitness professional if you're unsure about any variation.

By incorporating these woodchopper variations into your routine, you can keep your core training dynamic and challenging, continually stimulating muscle growth and improving your overall core strength, stability, and power. Remember, consistency and proper technique are key to unlocking the full potential of this versatile exercise and reaping its numerous benefits.

Common Mistakes in the Woodchopper Exercise and How to Correct Them

The woodchopper exercise, while seemingly straightforward, requires attention to detail to maximize its effectiveness and minimize the risk of injury. Here, we shed light on common mistakes that can hinder your progress and offer solutions to help you perform the woodchopper with optimal form.

Mistake #1: Improper Spine Position:

- **Incorrect:** Rounding your back or arching your lower back throughout the movement puts undue strain on your spine and increases the risk of injury.
- **Correction:** Maintain a neutral spine throughout the exercise. Imagine a straight line running from your head down your spine. Engage your core to maintain this

neutral position, keeping your back straight and avoiding excessive curvature.

Mistake #2: Lack of Core Engagement:

- **Incorrect:** Letting your core become loose and disengaged weakens the foundation of the movement and reduces its effectiveness.
- **Correction:** Consciously engage your core muscles throughout the entire exercise. Draw your belly button slightly inwards as you perform the movement, maintaining a tight and stable core.

Mistake #3: Arm Dominating the Movement:

- **Incorrect:** Relying primarily on your arm strength to lift the weight reduces the core's involvement and compromises the exercise's purpose.
- **Correction:** Initiating the movement with your core rotation is crucial. Think of your torso twisting and chopping the wood,

while your arms simply guide the weight along the movement path.

Mistake #4: Incorrect Shoulder Position:

- **Incorrect:** Shrugging your shoulders or allowing them to round forward during the movement can lead to shoulder pain and instability.
- **Correction:** Maintain a proud chest and keep your shoulders down and back throughout the exercise. Engage your shoulder blades to maintain proper posture and stability.

Mistake #5: Using Momentum Instead of Control:

- **Incorrect:** Swinging or jerking the weight with momentum can compromise form and increase the risk of injury.
- **Correction:** Perform the exercise in a controlled and deliberate manner. Focus on smoothly rotating your torso and

chopping the weight upwards, using your core muscles to control the movement.

Mistake #6: Weight Selection Beyond Your Capacity:

- **Incorrect:** Using a weight that is too heavy can lead to poor form and potentially result in injury.
- **Correction:** Start with a weight that allows you to maintain proper form throughout the entire exercise range of motion. Gradually increase the weight as your strength improves.

Mistake #7: Ignoring Breathing:

- **Incorrect:** Holding your breath during the exercise can increase blood pressure and hinder performance.
- **Correction:** Breathe naturally throughout the exercise. Exhale as you lift the weight and inhale as you lower it.

Additional Tips:

- Warm up your core and surrounding muscles before performing the woodchopper exercise.
- Maintain a full range of motion in your torso rotation while keeping your core engaged.
- Don't be afraid to seek guidance from a certified trainer or fitness professional to ensure you're performing the exercise with proper form.

By recognizing and correcting these common mistakes, you can ensure that your woodchopper exercise is not only effective but also safe and enjoyable. Remember, consistency and proper technique are key to reaping the numerous benefits of this exercise and building a strong, functional core.

Woodchopper Progressions and Regressions

Tailoring the Exercise to Your Fitness Level

The woodchopper exercise, a dynamic core movement, offers a wealth of benefits for individuals across various fitness levels. However, the key to maximizing its effectiveness and minimizing the risk of injury lies in **adapting the exercise to your individual needs and capabilities**. This is where progressions and regressions come into play, allowing you to modify the exercise difficulty to match your current fitness level.

Understanding Progressions and Regressions:

- **Progressions:** These are modifications that **increase the difficulty** of the exercise. As you get stronger, progressing the exercise allows you to continue challenging your core and promoting muscle growth.

- **Regressions:** These are modifications that **decrease the difficulty** of the exercise. This is crucial for beginners, individuals recovering from injuries, or those with limitations, allowing them to participate safely and effectively while building their core strength.

Progressions for Advanced Individuals:

- **Increase Weight:** Once you can comfortably perform the woodchopper with proper form using your bodyweight or a light weight, gradually increase the weight by using heavier dumbbells, kettlebells, or barbells. Start with a weight that allows you to maintain good form for all repetitions.
- **Single-Leg Woodchopper:** This variation adds a balance challenge and further engages your core stabilizers. Perform the woodchopper while standing on one leg,

ensuring proper form and core engagement throughout the movement.

- **Cable Woodchopper with Variations:** Utilize the cable machine for smooth resistance and explore different grip positions (neutral grip, wide grip) or cable attachments (rope attachment, stirrup attachment) to challenge your core from various angles.

Regressions for Beginners and Individuals with Limitations:

- **Bodyweight Woodchopper:** This is the most basic version of the exercise, ideal for beginners or those new to the movement. It allows you to focus on mastering the proper form and core engagement without the added weight of a dumbbell.
- **Medicine Ball Woodchopper with Lighter Ball:** Utilize a lighter medicine ball to decrease the weight and difficulty of the exercise. This allows you to focus on the rotational movement and core

engagement while adapting to the exercise.

- **Assisted Woodchopper:** Use a cable machine or resistance band with light resistance to provide some support while you perform the movement. This can be helpful for individuals with limitations or those recovering from injuries.
- **Partial Range of Motion:** If full range of motion is initially challenging, perform the woodchopper with a shorter range of motion, gradually increasing it as your strength and flexibility improve.

Additional Tips:

- **Focus on form over weight:** Always prioritize proper form over using a heavier weight. It's better to perform the exercise with good form and lighter weight than to sacrifice form for heavier weight.
- **Listen to your body:** It's crucial to listen to your body and stop if you experience any pain or discomfort. Consult a

healthcare professional if you have any concerns about modifying the exercise.

- **Seek professional guidance:** A certified trainer or fitness professional can help you choose the most appropriate progressions or regressions based on your individual needs and goals, ensuring you perform the exercise safely and effectively.

By understanding and utilizing progressions and regressions, you can tailor the woodchopper exercise to your specific fitness level, allowing you to progress safely and effectively on your journey towards a strong and functional core. Remember, consistency, proper technique, and adapting the exercise to your capabilities are key to reaping the full benefits of this versatile exercise.

Chapter 3

Part 3

Building Your Woodchopper Ab challenge

Sample Woodchopper Ab Workouts for Different Goals

The woodchopper exercise, renowned for its ability to sculpt a strong and functional core, can be incorporated into various workout routines to cater to diverse fitness goals. Here, we present several sample workouts featuring the woodchopper, tailored to specific objectives:

Goal: Build Core Strength and Stability

This workout focuses on building foundational core strength and stability by utilizing bodyweight variations and moderate repetitions.

Warm-up: 5-minute light cardio (jumping jacks, jogging in place) and dynamic stretches (arm circles, torso twists).

- **Bodyweight Woodchopper:** 3 sets of 12-15 repetitions per side
- **Plank:** 3 sets of 30-60 seconds hold
- **Bird-Dog:** 3 sets of 10-12 repetitions per side

Goal: Improve Core Endurance and Power

This workout emphasizes core endurance and power transfer by utilizing moderate weight and higher repetitions.

Warm-up: As above.

- **Cable Woodchopper (medium weight):** 3 sets of 15-20 repetitions per side
- **Russian Twist with Medicine Ball:** 3 sets of 12-15 repetitions per side
- **Anti-Rotational Press:** 3 sets of 10-12 repetitions per side

Goal: Sculpt a Defined Midsection

This workout combines the woodchopper with other core exercises that target different core muscles, promoting a more defined midsection.

Warm-up: As above.

- **Dumbbell Woodchopper (moderate weight):** 3 sets of 10-12 repetitions per side
- **Side Plank:** 3 sets of 30-60 seconds hold per side
- **Hanging Leg Raise:** 3 sets of 10-12 repetitions

Goal: Challenge Your Balance and Coordination

This workout integrates single-leg variations and other exercises that challenge your balance and coordination, enhancing core stability.

Warm-up: As above.

- **Single-Leg Woodchopper (bodyweight):** 3 sets of 8-10 repetitions per side
- **Single-Leg Deadlift:** 3 sets of 10-12 repetitions per side
- **Bosu Ball Plank:** 3 sets of 30-60 seconds hold

Cool-down: 5-minute static stretches (quad stretch, hamstring stretch, chest stretch).

Remember:

- These are just sample workouts; adjust the sets, repetitions, weight, and rest periods based on your individual fitness level and goals.
- Always prioritize proper form over weight or speed.
- Ensure proper rest (30-60 seconds) between sets and allow for adequate recovery days between workouts.
- Consult a certified trainer or fitness professional for personalized guidance and exercise modifications if needed.

By incorporating the woodchopper exercise into your routine and considering these sample workouts, you can effectively target your desired core goals, whether building strength and endurance, enhancing definition, or improving balance and coordination. Remember, consistency, proper technique, and tailoring the exercise to your capabilities are key to unlocking the full potential of the woodchopper and achieving a strong and functional core.

Structuring Your Woodchopper Ab Workouts

A Guide to Optimal Effectiveness

The woodchopper exercise, lauded for its ability to sculpt a strong and functional core, can be seamlessly integrated into various workout routines to cater to diverse fitness goals. However, to truly unlock its potential, **structured planning** is key. Here, we delve into the essential elements of structuring your woodchopper ab workouts for optimal effectiveness.

Understanding Your Goals:

The foundation of structuring your workout lies in **defining your specific goals**. Are you aiming to:

- **Build foundational core strength and stability?**
- **Improve core endurance and power transfer?**
- **Sculpt a defined midsection?**
- **Challenge your balance and coordination?**

Identifying your goals will guide you in selecting appropriate exercises and tailoring your workout parameters.

Planning Your Workout:

Once you've identified your goals, the planning phase begins. Consider the following elements:

- **Frequency:** Aim for 2-3 core workouts per week, spaced with adequate rest days for recovery.
- **Sets and Repetitions:**
    - **Strength and stability:** 3 sets of 8-12 repetitions.
    - **Endurance and power:** 3 sets of 15-20 repetitions.

- o **Definition:** 3 sets of 10-12 repetitions.
- **Rest:** Allow 30-60 seconds rest between sets to maintain intensity while facilitating recovery.
- **Progression:** Gradually increase weight, reps, or sets as you progress to avoid plateaus.
- **Warm-up and Cool-down:** Include a 5-minute light cardio and dynamic stretching warm-up and a 5-minute static stretching cool-down for optimal preparation and recovery.

Building Your Workout:

- **Selection of Exercises:** Choose exercises that complement the woodchopper and target different aspects of your core. Consider planks, side planks, hanging leg raises, and Russian twists for a well-rounded workout.
- **The Woodchopper's Role:**
  - o **Strength and stability:** Utilize bodyweight or lighter weight

variations for 3 sets of 8-12 repetitions per side.

- **Endurance and power:** Use moderate weight and aim for 3 sets of 15-20 repetitions per side.
- **Definition:** Integrate the woodchopper with other core exercises that target different regions, performing 3 sets of 10-12 repetitions per side.
- **Balance and coordination:** Utilize single-leg variations of the woodchopper and incorporate exercises like single-leg deadlifts and Bosu ball planks for 3 sets of 8-10 repetitions per side.

- **Sequencing:** Arrange exercises strategically. Start with compound exercises like the woodchopper, followed by isolation exercises like hanging leg raises, and conclude with exercises that challenge balance and coordination, like single-leg deadlifts.

Additional Tips:

- **Focus on form over weight:** Prioritize proper technique for safe and effective execution.
- **Listen to your body:** Adjust weight, repetitions, and rest periods based on your individual needs and avoid pushing yourself to the point of pain.
- **Seek professional guidance:** A certified trainer or fitness professional can help design a personalized workout plan tailored to your specific goals and limitations.

By understanding your goals, planning your workouts strategically, and incorporating these elements, you can structure woodchopper ab workouts that are effective, safe, and enjoyable. Remember, consistency, proper technique, and mindful planning are key to unlocking the full potential of this versatile exercise and achieving a strong, functional core.

Integrating the Woodchopper into Your Overall Fitness Routine

The woodchopper exercise, often associated solely with core training, has the potential to be a valuable asset in your **overall fitness routine**. Its dynamic nature and ability to engage various muscle groups make it a versatile tool that can enhance your workouts in several ways:

1. Core Strength and Stability:

- **Primary Target:** The woodchopper primarily targets your **obliques**, the muscles on the sides of your torso responsible for rotation and spinal stabilization.
- **Additional Benefits:** It also engages your **rectus abdominis (six-pack)** for stability and the **lower back muscles** to maintain proper posture throughout the movement. This comprehensive engagement strengthens your core, improving stability,

posture, and reducing the risk of lower back pain.

2. Rotational Power and Control:

- **Rotational Movement:** The woodchopper mimics rotational movements found in various sports and everyday activities, such as throwing, swinging, and chopping.
- **Power Transfer:** By strengthening the muscles responsible for rotation, the woodchopper improves your ability to transfer power efficiently, enhancing performance in activities that require rotational power.

3. Improved Balance and Coordination:

- **Dynamic Exercise:** The woodchopper involves coordinated movement of your upper and lower body while maintaining a stable core.
- **Balance Challenge:** This dynamic nature challenges your balance and coordination,

which are crucial for various physical activities and overall well-being.

4. Increased Metabolic Demand:

- **Full-Body Engagement:** The woodchopper engages multiple muscle groups simultaneously, leading to a higher metabolic demand compared to isolation exercises.
- **Calorie Burning:** This increased metabolic demand translates to burning more calories during your workout, contributing to weight management and overall fitness goals.

Integrating the Woodchopper:

1. As a Warm-up:

- **Light Weight or Bodyweight:** Perform a few sets of the woodchopper with light weight or bodyweight to activate your core and prepare your body for the workout.

2. As a Main Exercise:

- **Multiple Sets and Variations:** Include 2-3 sets of 8-15 repetitions of the woodchopper, incorporating variations like cable woodchopper, medicine ball woodchopper, or single-leg woodchopper to target different aspects of core strength and challenge yourself throughout the workout.

3. As a Finisher:

- **High-Intensity Sets:** Perform 1-2 sets of the woodchopper with higher intensity (increased weight or faster tempo) to challenge your core and test your endurance at the end of your workout.

Remember:

- **Prioritize Form:** Focus on proper form over weight to maximize effectiveness and prevent injury. Keep your core engaged, back straight, and rotate through your torso rather than your lower back.

- **Progression:** Gradually increase weight, sets, or repetitions as you get stronger to maintain a challenge and promote continuous improvement.
- **Listen to Your Body:** Take rest days when needed and avoid exceeding your limits to prevent overtraining and potential injury.

The woodchopper, when integrated strategically, can be a valuable addition to your fitness routine, offering a multitude of benefits beyond core strength. Its versatility and effectiveness make it a worthy tool for sculpting a well-rounded physique and enhancing your overall fitness.

Warming Up and Cooling Down for Peak Ab Workouts

Ensuring proper warm-up and cool-down routines is crucial for maximizing the effectiveness and safety of your ab workouts, including those incorporating the woodchopper exercise. Here's a breakdown of essential warm-up and cool-down strategies:

Warm-Up (5-10 Minutes):

- **Goal:** Increase blood flow, elevate core temperature, and prepare your muscles for movement.
- **Activities:**
    - **Light cardio:** 5 minutes of jumping jacks, jogging in place, or jumping rope to elevate your heart rate and blood flow.
    - **Dynamic stretches:** Focus on stretches that mimic the movements you'll perform in your workout. Include:

- **Arm circles (forward and backward):** 10-12 repetitions each direction.
- **Torso twists:** 10-12 repetitions each direction.
- **Leg swings (front and back):** 10-12 repetitions each leg.
- **High knees and butt kicks:** 30 seconds each.

Cool-Down (5-10 Minutes):

- **Goal:** Gradually decrease heart rate, improve flexibility, and promote muscle recovery.
- **Activities:**
  - **Light cardio:** 3-5 minutes of walking or light jogging.
  - **Static stretches:** Hold each stretch for 30-60 seconds, focusing on major muscle groups engaged during your workout, including:

- **Hamstring stretch:** Sit with legs extended, reach for your toes, keeping your back straight.
- **Quad stretch:** Stand on one leg, pull your other foot towards your glutes while maintaining balance.
- **Chest stretch:** Clasp your hands behind your back and gently push your chest forward.
- **Lower back stretch:** Lie on your back with knees bent, hug your knees to your chest and hold.

Additional Tips:

- **Listen to your body:** Adjust the intensity and duration of your warm-up and cool-down based on your individual needs and the intensity of your workout.

- **Stay hydrated:** Drink plenty of water throughout your workout and during your cool-down to aid recovery.
- **Don't skip the cool-down:** While it might be tempting to skip the cool-down, it's essential for reducing muscle soreness and improving flexibility.

By incorporating these warm-up and cool-down routines into your ab workouts, you'll prepare your body for optimal performance, minimize the risk of injury, and promote faster recovery, allowing you to reap the full benefits of your training. Remember, consistency with both your workout routines and these preparatory measures is key to achieving your fitness goals.

Part 4

Chapter 4

Beyond the Woodchopper: Additional Core Exercises

Complementary Exercises for Core Strength and Stability

The woodchopper exercise, renowned for its ability to engage and strengthen your core, is a valuable tool in your core training arsenal. However, to truly build a strong and stable core, it's crucial to incorporate a **diverse range of complementary exercises**. This ensures you target different core muscles and movement patterns, leading to well-rounded core development. Here, we explore various exercises that effectively complement the woodchopper, catering to different muscle groups and training goals:

Targeting Different Core Muscles:

- **Plank Variations:** Engage your entire core with variations like the high plank (on hands), low plank (on forearms), side plank (on one side), and hollow body hold. These variations challenge different stabilizing muscles and offer progression options.
- **Bird-Dog:** This exercise emphasizes core stability and coordination by simultaneously engaging your core, glutes, and shoulders. Start on all fours, extend one arm and the opposite leg while maintaining a flat back.
- **Anti-Rotational Press:** Utilize cables or resistance bands to perform this exercise, which challenges your core's ability to resist rotation. This is crucial for activities like throwing and preventing lower back pain.
- **Dead Bug:** This exercise isolates your deep core muscles, promoting stability and proper spine alignment. Lie on your

back with knees bent and feet flat on the floor. Extend one arm and the opposite leg while maintaining a neutral spine and keeping your lower back pressed into the ground.

Exercises for Specific Training Goals:

- **Strength and Stability:**
    - **Deadlift:** This compound exercise, while primarily targeting your posterior chain, also significantly engages your core for stability and proper form.
    - **Squat:** Similar to the deadlift, squats engage your core to maintain stability throughout the movement.
- **Endurance and Power:**
    - **Russian Twist:** This exercise challenges your core with rotational movements, improving core endurance and power transfer. Sit on the floor with knees bent and feet flat, rotate your torso from side

to side while maintaining a slightly leaned-back position.

- **Medicine Ball Slams:** This dynamic exercise is a great way to challenge your core and improve power transfer. Stand with feet shoulder-width apart, hold a medicine ball overhead, and slam it forcefully down onto the ground in front of you.

- **Balance and Coordination:**
  - **Single-leg Deadlift:** This variation of the deadlift adds a balance challenge, forcing your core to work harder for stability. Stand on one leg, hinge forward while keeping your back straight, and reach towards the ground with your other hand.
  - **Bosu Ball Plank:** Perform a regular plank position on a Bosu ball, adding an element of instability that requires your core to work overtime to maintain balance.

Integration with Woodchopper Workouts:

The woodchopper can be effectively combined with these complementary exercises to create well-rounded core workouts. Here are some sample structures:

Sample Workout 1: Core Strength and Stability

- Warm-up (5 minutes)
- Woodchopper (bodyweight): 3 sets of 10-12 repetitions per side
- Plank (high or low): 3 sets of 30-60 seconds hold
- Bird-Dog: 3 sets of 8-10 repetitions per side
- Deadlift (light weight): 3 sets of 8-12 repetitions
- Cool-down (5 minutes)

Sample Workout 2: Core Endurance and Power

- Warm-up (5 minutes)

- Woodchopper (moderate weight): 3 sets of 15-20 repetitions per side
- Russian Twist with medicine ball: 3 sets of 12-15 repetitions per side
- Medicine Ball Slams: 3 sets of 10-12 repetitions
- Squat: 3 sets of 12-15 repetitions
- Cool-down (5 minutes)

Remember:

- These are just examples; adjust exercises, sets, repetitions, and weight based on your fitness level and goals.
- Prioritize proper form over weight or speed.
- Allow adequate rest between sets and workouts for optimal recovery.
- Seek guidance from a certified trainer or fitness professional for personalized exercise selection and challenge ming.

By incorporating these complementary exercises and the woodchopper into your routine, you can create a comprehensive core training challenge that addresses different muscle groups, training goals, and movement patterns. Remember, consistency, proper technique, and a well-rounded approach are key to achieving a strong, stable, and functional core.

Building a Well-Rounded Core Training challenge :

A strong and functional core is the foundation for a healthy body, improving posture, stability, performance in various activities, and even reducing the risk of injuries. While exercises like the woodchopper offer significant benefits, building a **well-rounded core training challenge** requires a strategic approach that encompasses various elements. This guide delves into the key aspects of creating an effective and comprehensive core training challenge .

Solidifying Your Foundation: Understanding Core Function

Before embarking on your core training journey, it's crucial to understand the **core's function**. Your core encompasses a group of muscles, including the:

- **Rectus abdominis (six-pack):** Provides stability and supports trunk flexion.

- **Obliques:** Assist with rotation, lateral flexion, and support the spine.
- **Transverse abdominis (deep core):** Provides stability and assists with breathing.
- **Lower back muscles:** Support the spine and aid in movement.

Goals and Needs: Identifying Your Objectives

The first step in building your challenge is defining your **specific goals**. Do you want to:

- **Build core strength and stability?**
- **Improve core endurance and power transfer?**
- **Develop a defined midsection?**
- **Enhance balance and coordination?**

Identifying your goals helps you choose exercises, sets, repetitions, and progression strategies tailored to your needs.

Selecting Exercises: A Diverse Arsenal

Building a Well-Rounded Core Training challenge

While the woodchopper is a valuable tool, relying solely on it limits your core development. A well-rounded challenge incorporates exercises that target different core muscles and movement patterns. Consider:

- **Compound exercises:** Engage multiple muscle groups, including planks, squats, deadlifts, and lunges. These exercises significantly challenge your core while strengthening other muscle groups.
- **Isolation exercises:** Target specific core muscles, including hanging leg raises, crunches, side planks, and bird-dogs. These exercises help refine core strength and definition.
- **Rotational exercises:** Challenge your core's ability to resist rotation, such as Russian twists, anti-rotational presses, and medicine ball throws. These exercises improve core stability and power transfer.

- **Balance and coordination exercises:** Engage your core to maintain stability in dynamic movements, such as single-leg exercises, Bosu ball exercises, and stability ball exercises.

Balancing Strength and Endurance:

- **Strength:** Aim for 3 sets of 8-12 repetitions with a weight that challenges you towards the end of the set.
- **Endurance:** Aim for 3 sets of 15-20 repetitions with moderate weight or bodyweight exercises.
- **Power:** Utilize explosive movements like medicine ball slams or jump squats with lighter weights for 3 sets of 8-12 repetitions.

Progression and Variation:

To avoid plateaus and continuously challenge your core, incorporate **progression** and **variation**:

- **Increase weight, sets, or repetitions** as you get stronger.
- **Modify exercises** to target different muscle groups or movement patterns.

Frequency and Rest:

- Aim for **2-3 core workouts per week**, spaced with **adequate rest days** (24-48 hours) for optimal recovery.
- Allow **30-60 seconds rest** between sets.

Warm-up and Cool-down:

- **Warm up** with 5 minutes of light cardio and dynamic stretches to prepare your muscles for movement.
- **Cool down** with 5 minutes of static stretches to improve flexibility and promote recovery.

Additional Tips:

- **Focus on form over weight:** Prioritize proper technique to avoid injury and maximize effectiveness.

- **Listen to your body:** Adjust intensity and rest based on your needs.
- **Seek professional guidance:** A certified trainer can customize a challenge to your specific goals and limitations.

Conclusion:

Building a well-rounded core training challenge requires a **combination of diverse exercises, targeted training goals, and strategic planning**. By incorporating the elements outlined above and remaining consistent, you can achieve a strong, functional core that enhances your overall health, performance, and well-being. Remember, a well-rounded approach, proper technique, and a focus on your individual needs are key to unlocking the full potential of your core training journey.

Sample Core Training challenge with Woodchopper Variations

This sample challenge incorporates the woodchopper exercise alongside various complementary exercises to create a well-rounded core workout routine. You can adjust the exercises, sets, repetitions, and rest periods based on your fitness level and goals.

Warm-up (5 minutes):

- Light cardio (jumping jacks, jogging in place, jumping rope)
- Dynamic stretches (arm circles, torso twists, leg swings)

Workout (30-45 minutes):

Round 1:

- **Woodchopper (bodyweight):** 3 sets of 12 repetitions per side

- **Plank (high or low):** 3 sets of 30 seconds hold

Round 2:

- **Single-leg deadlift (bodyweight):** 3 sets of 10 repetitions per leg
- **Bird-dog:** 3 sets of 8 repetitions per side

Round 3:

- **Cable woodchopper (moderate weight):** 3 sets of 15 repetitions per side
- **Russian twist with medicine ball:** 3 sets of 12 repetitions per side

Cool-down (5 minutes):

- Static stretches (hamstring stretch, quad stretch, chest stretch, lower back stretch)

Progression:

- As you get stronger, you can progress by:
    - Increasing the weight used in the woodchopper and cable woodchopper exercises.

- ○ Performing more repetitions or sets of each exercise.
  - ○ Shortening the rest periods between sets.
- You can also progress by adding more challenging variations of the exercises, such as:
  - ○ Using a heavier weight or kettlebell for the woodchopper and cable woodchopper.
  - ○ Performing the woodchopper on a stability ball.
  - ○ Adding a jump to the single-leg deadlift.

Additional Notes:

- This is just a sample challenge , and you may need to adjust it based on your individual needs and goals.
- It's important to listen to your body and take rest days when needed.
- Always consult with a doctor or certified trainer before starting any new exercise challenge .

Remember, consistency, proper form, and a well-rounded approach are key to achieving a strong and functional core.

Part 5: Nutrition and Lifestyle Tips for Core Development

Chapter 5

Building a Strong Core

The Role of Nutrition in Building a Strong Core

Building a strong and functional core requires a **two-pronged approach**: **strategic training and proper nutrition**. While exercises like the woodchopper are crucial, the food you consume plays an equally vital role in providing the building blocks and fuel your core muscles need to develop and thrive. Here's how nutrition contributes to a strong core:

Energy for Training:

- **Carbohydrates:** Complex carbohydrates, like whole grains, fruits, and vegetables, provide sustained energy to power your core workouts. They are broken down into glucose, the primary fuel source for your muscles.

- **Protein:** Protein is essential for building and repairing muscle tissue, including your core muscles. Aim for protein sources like lean meats, poultry, fish, eggs, legumes, and dairy products.

Muscle Recovery and Growth:

- **Protein:** Post-workout protein intake is crucial for repairing and rebuilding muscle fibers damaged during exercise, promoting core muscle growth and strength.
- **Healthy fats:** Include healthy fats, like those found in avocados, nuts, seeds, and olive oil, in your diet. These fats contribute to hormone production, regulate inflammation, and aid in nutrient absorption, supporting overall muscle recovery and health.

Overall Core Health and Function:

- **Micronutrients:** Vitamins and minerals play various roles in core health and function. Vitamin D promotes calcium absorption, crucial for bone health and core stability. Vitamin C aids in collagen production, essential for connective tissue health and overall core support.
- **Hydration:** Adequate hydration is essential for optimal muscle function and recovery. Aim to drink plenty of water throughout the day and during your workouts to stay hydrated and support core performance.

Nutritional Tips for a Strong Core:

- **Eat a balanced diet:** Include a variety of fruits, vegetables, whole grains, lean protein sources, and healthy fats in your daily meals.
- **Focus on whole foods:** Prioritize whole, unprocessed foods over sugary drinks and processed snacks.
- **Time your meals strategically:** Consume a well-balanced pre-workout meal rich in

complex carbohydrates and protein to fuel your workout. Opt for a protein-rich post-workout meal to aid muscle recovery.

- **Stay hydrated:** Drink plenty of water throughout the day to stay hydrated and support core function.
- **Seek guidance:** Consult a registered dietitian or nutritionist for personalized dietary advice tailored to your specific fitness goals and needs.

Remember, **nutrition is a cornerstone of building a strong core**. By providing your body with the right fuel and nutrients, you can significantly enhance the effectiveness of your core training challenge and achieve optimal results. Consistent and well-planned nutrition, combined with dedicated training, will pave the way for a strong, functional core that supports your overall health and well-being.

Lifestyle Habits for a Strong and Healthy Core

While dedicated core training and proper nutrition are essential for building a strong core, a **holistic approach** incorporating various **lifestyle habits** can further optimize your core health and stability. These habits, when implemented consistently, create a supportive environment for your core to flourish:

1. Maintaining Good Posture:

- **Practice good posture throughout the day:** Be mindful of your posture while sitting, standing, and walking. Keep your spine straight, shoulders back and down, and core engaged.
- **Utilize ergonomic tools:** Use ergonomic chairs, desks, and monitors to promote proper posture and reduce strain on your core muscles.

- **Perform posture-focused exercises:** Include exercises like wall slides, planks with scapular retraction, and chin tucks in your routine to strengthen muscles that support good posture.

2. Prioritizing Quality Sleep:

- **Aim for 7-8 hours of sleep per night:** Adequate sleep allows your body to repair and rebuild tissues, including your core muscles, promoting optimal recovery and core health.
- **Establish a consistent sleep schedule:** Go to bed and wake up at similar times each day, even on weekends, to regulate your sleep-wake cycle and improve sleep quality.
- **Create a relaxing bedtime routine:** This could include taking a warm bath, reading a book, or practicing relaxation techniques like deep breathing or meditation before bed to promote restful sleep.

3. Managing Stress Effectively:

- **Identify and manage stress factors:** Chronic stress can negatively impact your core health by increasing cortisol levels, which can lead to muscle breakdown and hinder muscle growth.
- **Incorporate stress-relieving activities:** Engage in activities that help you manage stress, such as yoga, meditation, deep breathing exercises, spending time in nature, or listening to calming music.
- **Maintain a healthy work-life balance:** Make time for activities you enjoy and that help you de-stress outside of work or school commitments.

4. Maintaining a Healthy Weight:

- **Eat a balanced and healthy diet:** A healthy diet rich in fruits, vegetables, whole grains, and lean protein sources helps maintain a healthy weight and reduces strain on your core muscles.
- **Engage in regular physical activity:** Aim for at least 150 minutes of moderate-intensity exercise or 75 minutes

of vigorous-intensity exercise per week. This not only helps manage weight but also strengthens your core muscles.

- **Consult a healthcare professional:** If you struggle with maintaining a healthy weight, consult a doctor or registered dietitian for personalized guidance and support.

5. Addressing Underlying Issues:

- **Seek professional help for chronic pain or discomfort:** If you experience chronic pain or discomfort in your core region, consult a healthcare professional to identify and address the underlying cause. This could involve physical therapy, medication, or lifestyle modifications.
- **Maintain regular checkups with your doctor:** Regular checkups with your doctor can help identify any potential health concerns that may impact your core health or overall well-being.

Remember: Consistency is key. By incorporating these lifestyle habits into your daily routine, you can create a supportive environment for your core to thrive and contribute to a strong, healthy core that underpins your overall well-being.

Recap and Final Thoughts

Cultivating a Comprehensive Approach to Core Strength

Throughout this discussion, we've delved into various aspects of building a strong and functional core, venturing beyond the realm of the woodchopper exercise. We've explored the importance of:

- **Understanding your goals:** Defining your core training goals is crucial for choosing appropriate exercises and tailoring your workout challenge .
- **Building a well-rounded challenge :** Incorporating diverse exercises targeting various core muscles and movement patterns is essential for comprehensive core development.
- **Proper form and technique:** Prioritizing proper form over weight or speed minimizes the risk of injury and maximizes the effectiveness of your training.

- **Progression and variation:** Continuously challenging your core with increased weight, repetitions, or variations prevents plateaus and keeps your workouts engaging.
- **Nutritional support:** Providing your body with the right fuel through balanced meals and proper hydration empowers optimal core function and recovery.
- **Supportive lifestyle habits:** Maintaining good posture, prioritizing quality sleep, managing stress, and maintaining a healthy weight create a foundation for optimal core health.

Final Thoughts:

Building a strong core is not a singular act but a **continuous journey** that requires dedication, consistency, and a **holistic approach**. By combining targeted exercises with proper nutrition, supportive lifestyle habits, and a focus on well-being, you can cultivate a strong and functional core that not only enhances your physical performance but also underpins your overall health and quality of life.

Remember, the path to a strong core is individual, and what works for someone else might not be the best approach for you. Listen to your body, seek guidance from qualified professionals, and adjust your strategies as needed. Embrace the journey, stay consistent, and celebrate every step forward as you build a core that empowers you to move with confidence and embrace a healthier, more fulfilling life.

Glossary of Terms

Core: A group of muscles in the torso that provide stability, support the spine, and aid in movement.

Core strength: The ability of the core muscles to generate force and support the body.

Core stability: The ability of the core muscles to maintain a neutral spine and control movement.

Functional core: A core that is strong and stable enough to support everyday activities and athletic performance.

Warm-up: A period of light cardio and dynamic stretches to prepare the body for exercise.

Cool-down: A period of static stretches to improve flexibility and promote recovery after exercise.

Compound exercise: An exercise that engages multiple muscle groups at the same time.

Isolation exercise: An exercise that targets a specific muscle group.

Rotational exercise: An exercise that challenges the core's ability to resist rotation.

Progression: Gradually increasing the difficulty of an exercise over time.

Rest: The time between sets of exercises to allow the muscles to recover.

Micronutrients: Vitamins and minerals essential for various bodily functions.

Posture: The position of the body when standing, sitting, or walking.

Ergonomic: Designed to provide comfort and minimize stress on the body.

Chronic stress: Long-term stress that can negatively impact physical and mental health.

Overall well-being: A state of physical, mental, and social health.

Sample Core Workout Log Sheet

This template provides a basic structure for recording your core workouts. You can customize it to fit your specific needs and preferences.

Date: [Date of Workout]

Warm-up: (List the warm-up activities you performed and the duration)

Workout:

Cool-down: (List the cool-down activities you performed and the duration)

Notes:

- You can add additional columns to your log sheet to track other information, such as the perceived exertion level on a scale of 1-10 (RPE), any modifications you made to the exercises, or how you felt overall after the workout.
- It is important to be honest and accurate when recording your workout information. This will help you track your progress over time and make adjustments to your challenge as needed.

Additional Tips:

- Consider using a different color pen for each exercise or set.
- Laminate your workout log sheet so you can reuse it.
- Download a workout log app on your phone or tablet.

Sample workout log sheet plan

Bonus

https://go.screenpal.com/watch/cZei1YVK7NW

Video link for tutorials